MommyHooray Presents:

Emotional Labor

The Quiet Work That Keeps Everything Running

by MommyHooray

MommyHooray Presents: Emotional Labor
by MommyHooray

Written and published under the pen name MommyHooray.
Illustrations created using digital illustration tools.

Printed in the United States of America.

ISBN: 978-1-972071-42-7

For more stories and updates, visit:
https://sites.google.com/view/mommyhooray

To the one who carries it all—
the thoughts, the plans, the feelings no one else sees.

I see you.
I see how much you hold,
how much you remember,
how much you give
without being asked.

Even on the days it feels invisible, it is not.
It matters. You matter.

This is for you.

With Googolplex Love,

MommyHooray ♡

Some work is loud.
You can see it pile up, measure it, check it off a list.

But some work is invisible.
It lives in the pauses,
in the remembering,
in the noticing before anyone asks.

It is the weight of keeping things running
without ever being told to.

It is emotional labor.

And if you've been carrying it—
this is for you.

You remember everything.
Appointments, preferences, moods,
the little things that hold a life together.

Not because you were told to—
but because no one else would.

You carry the details that keep life moving,
the small things that are never really small.

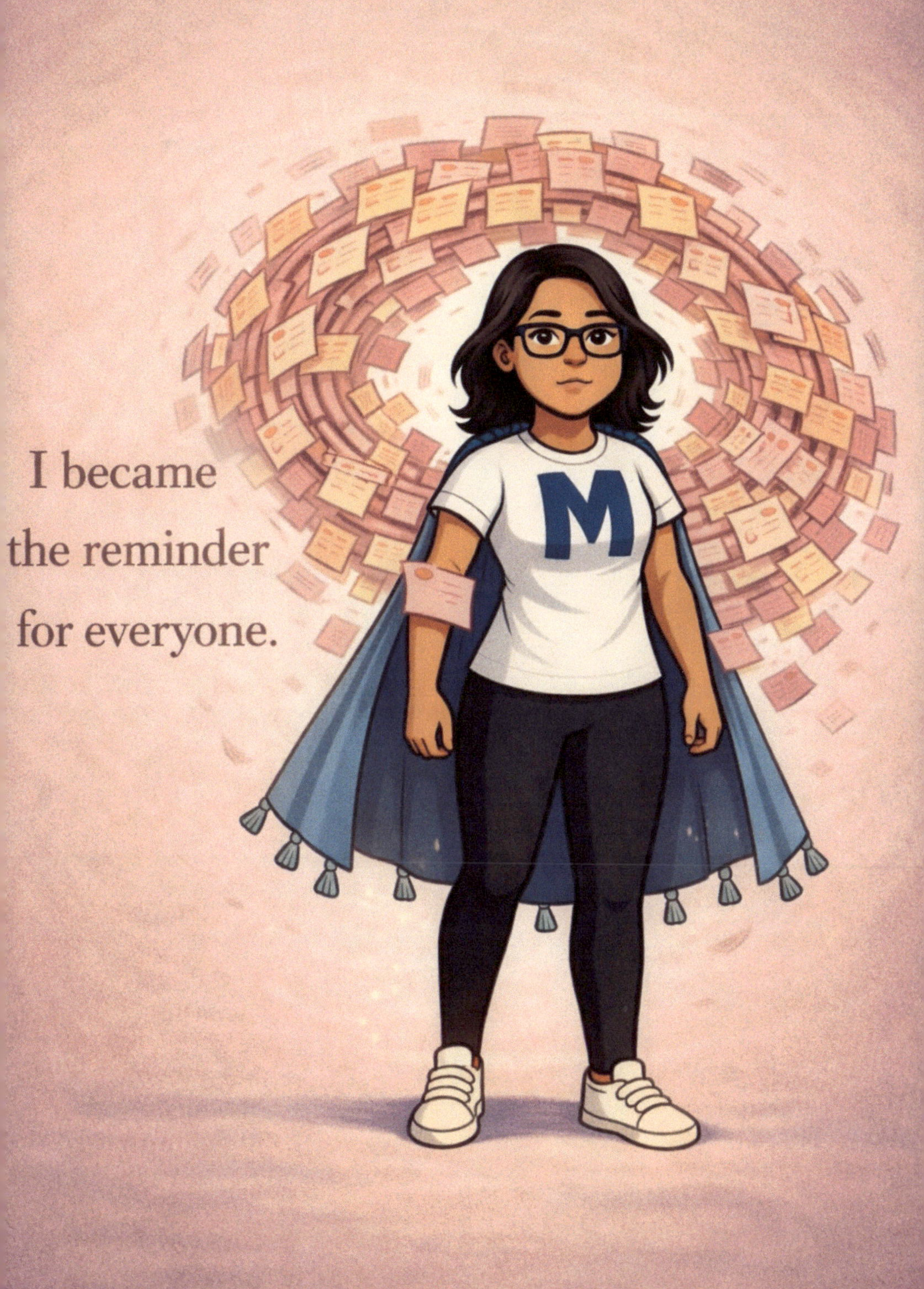

I became
the reminder
for everyone.

You notice the shift in tone.
The silence that means something is wrong.
The tension before it becomes a problem.

You adjust before anyone asks you to.

You step in quietly, holding things together
before they fall apart.

That isn't small.
That's care.

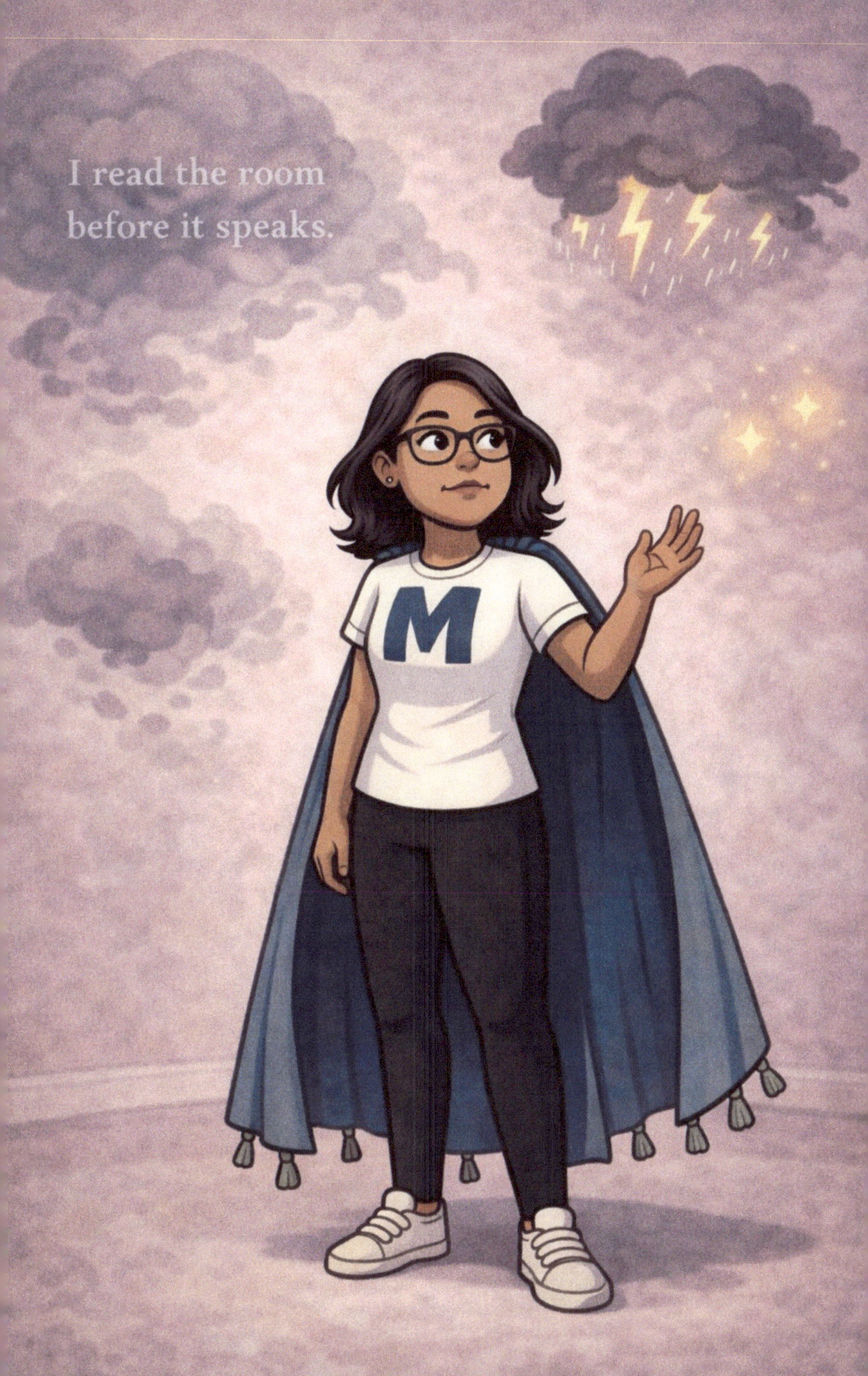
I read the room
before it speaks.
M

You plan ahead.
Not just for today—
but for what might happen tomorrow.

You carry the “just in case.”
The quiet preparation.
The unseen safety net.

Always thinking one step forward,
so everyone else can stay right where they are.

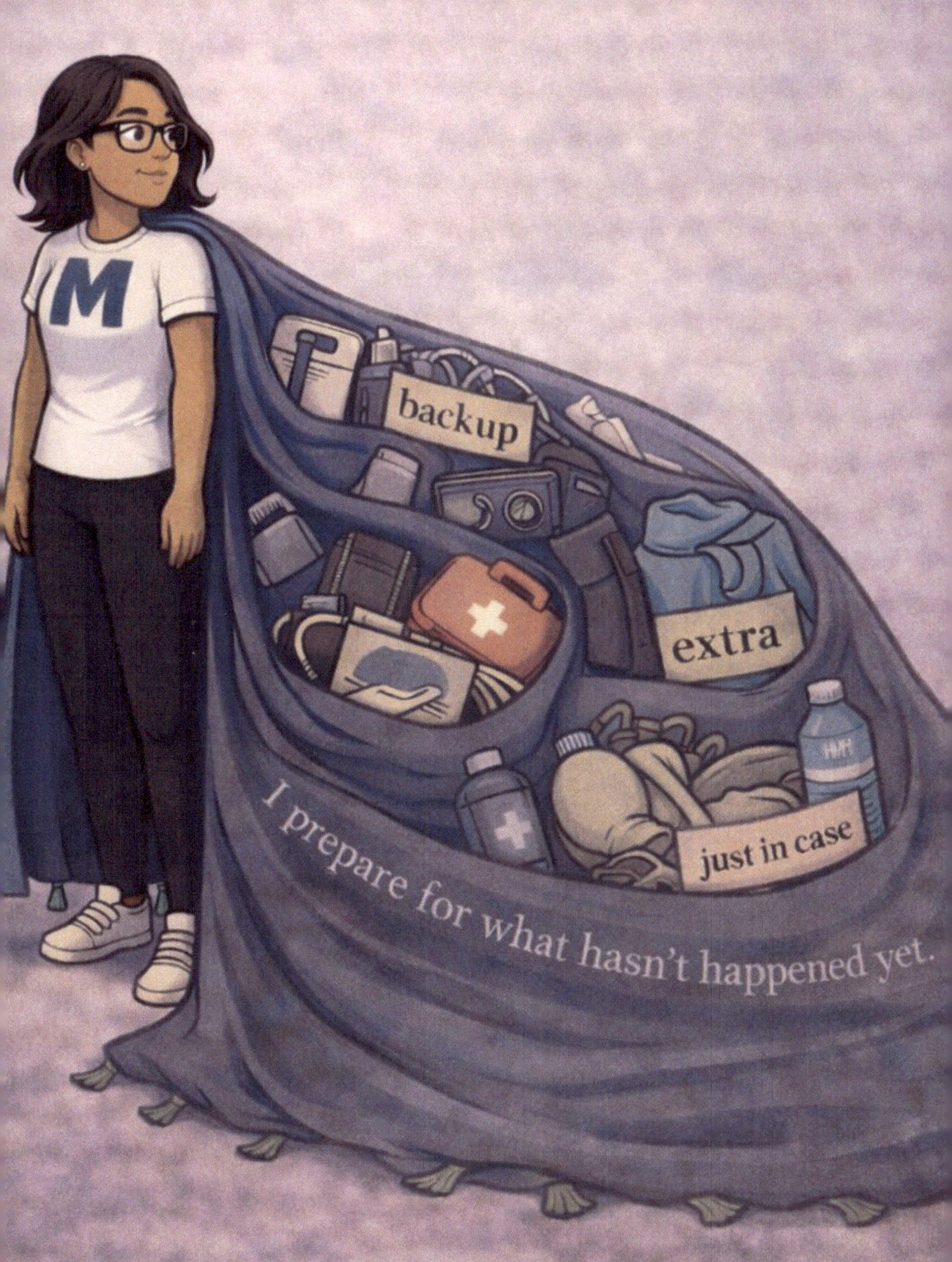
backup
extra
just in case
I prepare for what hasn't happened yet.

You smooth things over.

Translate feelings.

Soften words.

Keep the peace.

Even when it costs you yours.

You hold the tension so others don't have to.

You carry the weight no one names.

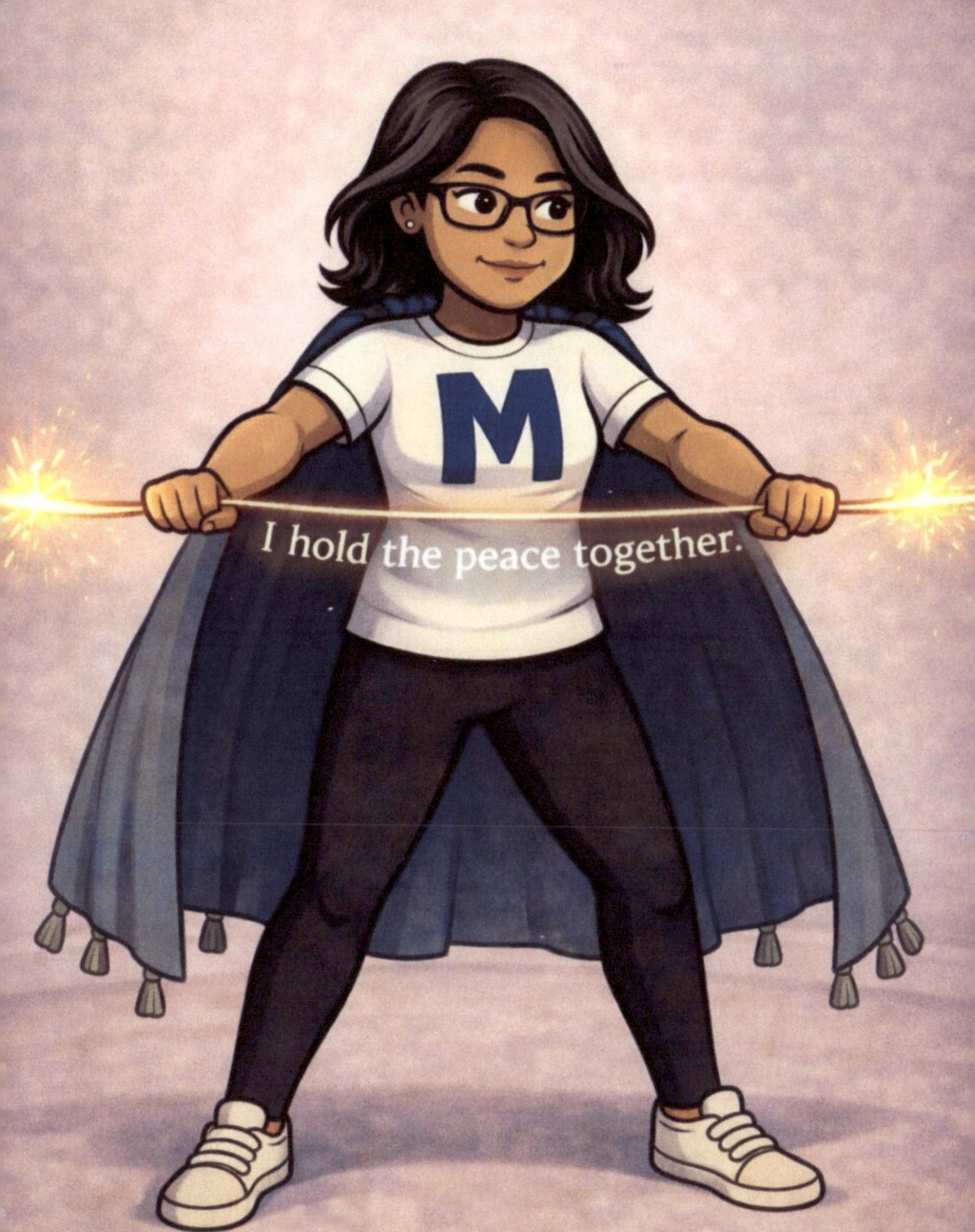
I hold the peace together.
M

Even after it's over,
the conversation stays with you.

You think it through again—
what you said, what you didn't,
what you wish you had done differently.

Because you care.

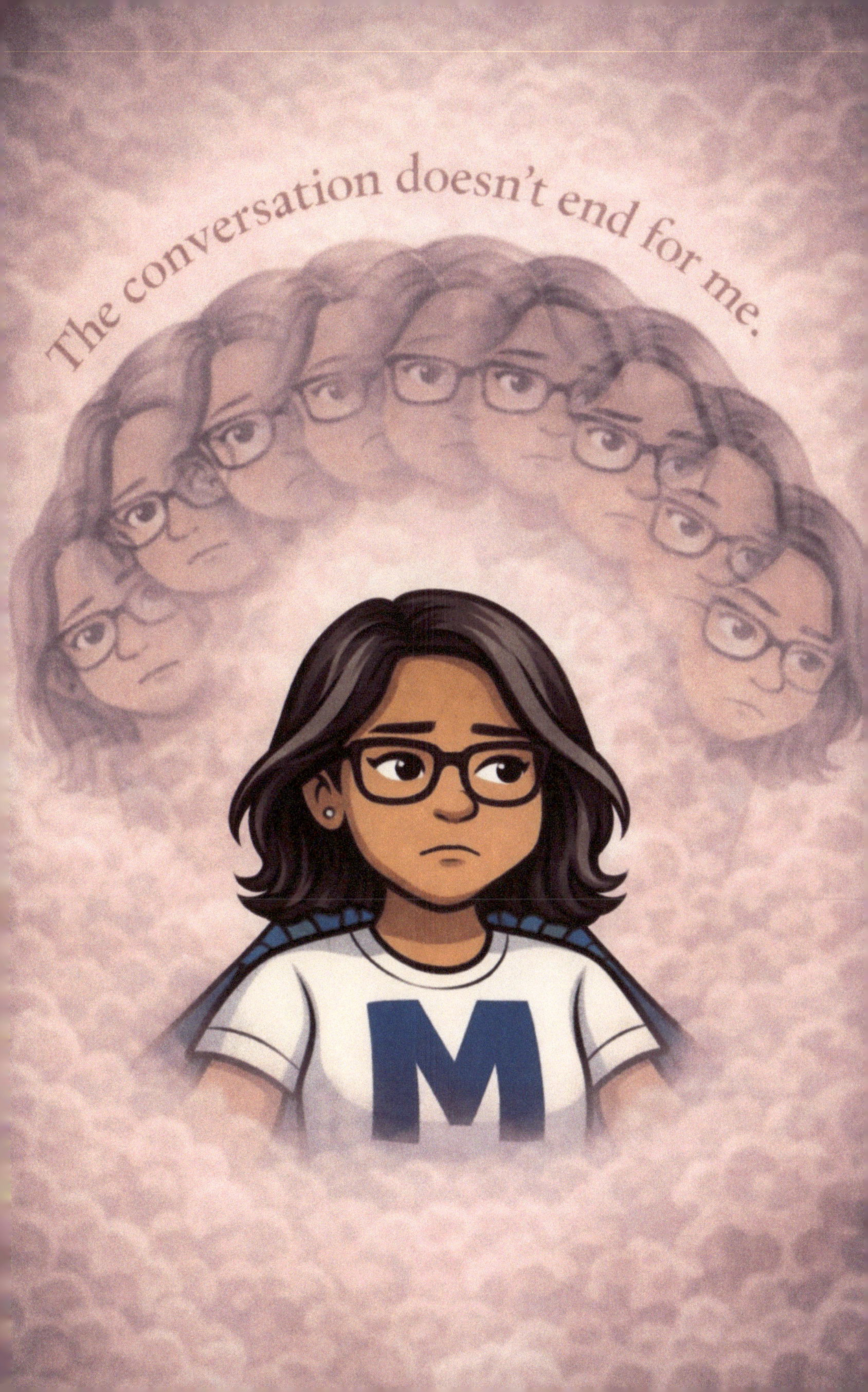

The conversation doesn't end for me.

You make things feel special.
Birthdays, holidays, the little moments in between.

You create magic—
even when you're tired.

Because you care.
Because you want it to feel meaningful.

And it does—because of you.

I create moments no one realizes I built.

You anticipate needs
before they are spoken.

Water before they're thirsty.
Comfort before they ask.

Because you're paying attention.
Because you care that deeply.

And that care shows up—every time.

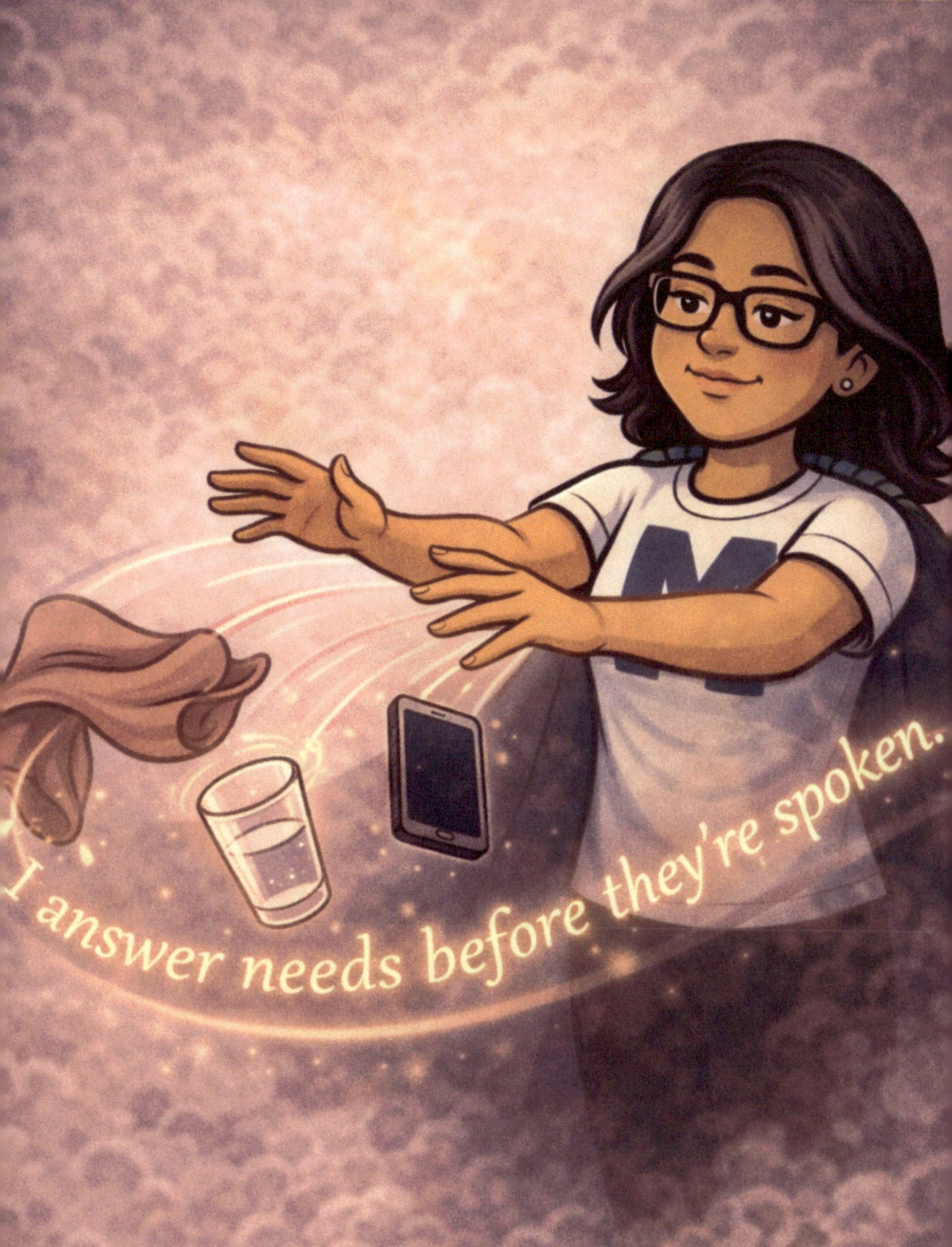
M
I answer needs before they're spoken.

You carry the emotional temperature
of everyone around you.

And somehow,
you're expected to stay steady.

Even when it feels like too much.

Even when no one asks how you're doing.

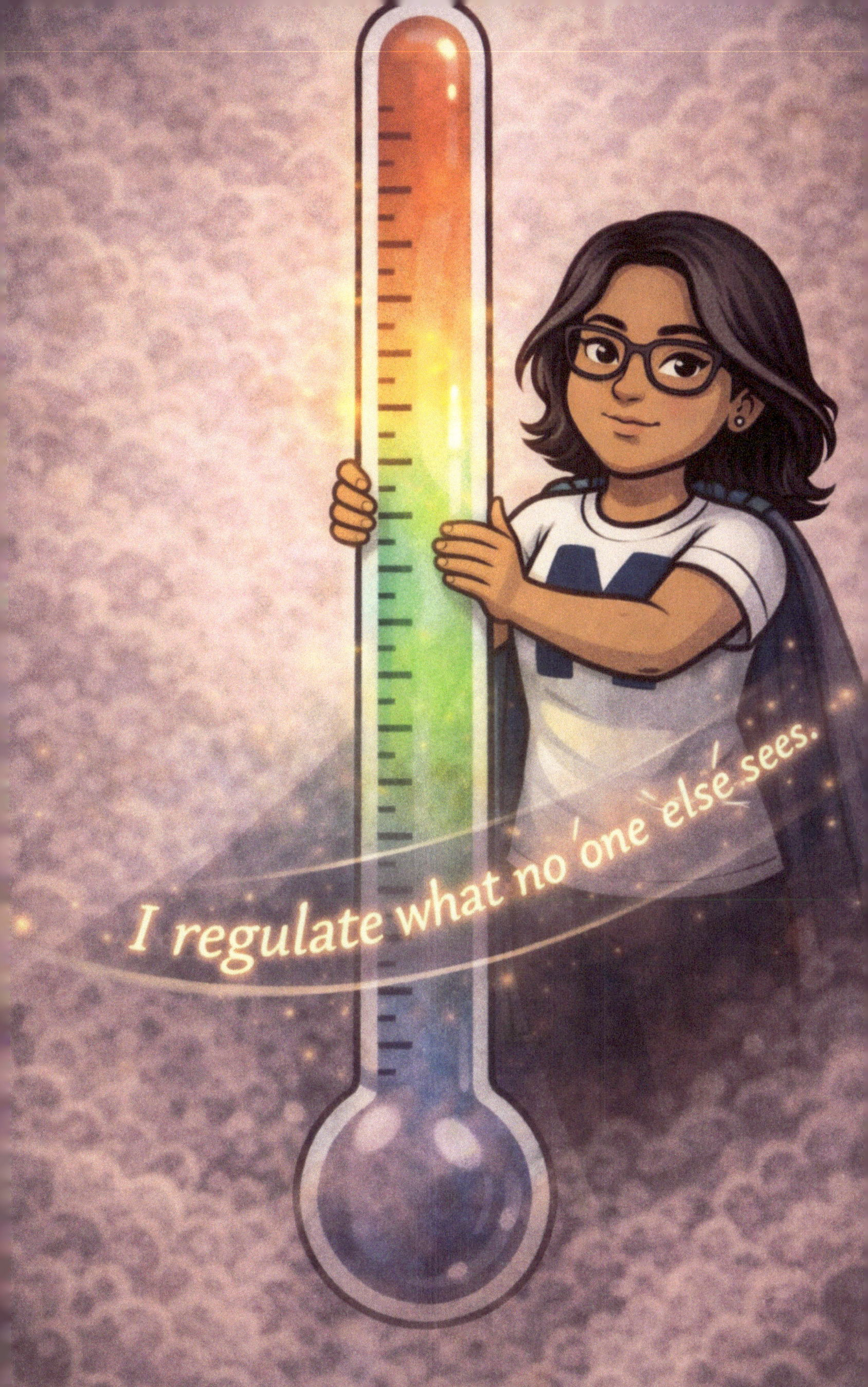
I regulate what no one else sees.

You check in.

You follow up.

You remember the small details.

Even when no one checks on you.

You give what you don't always receive.

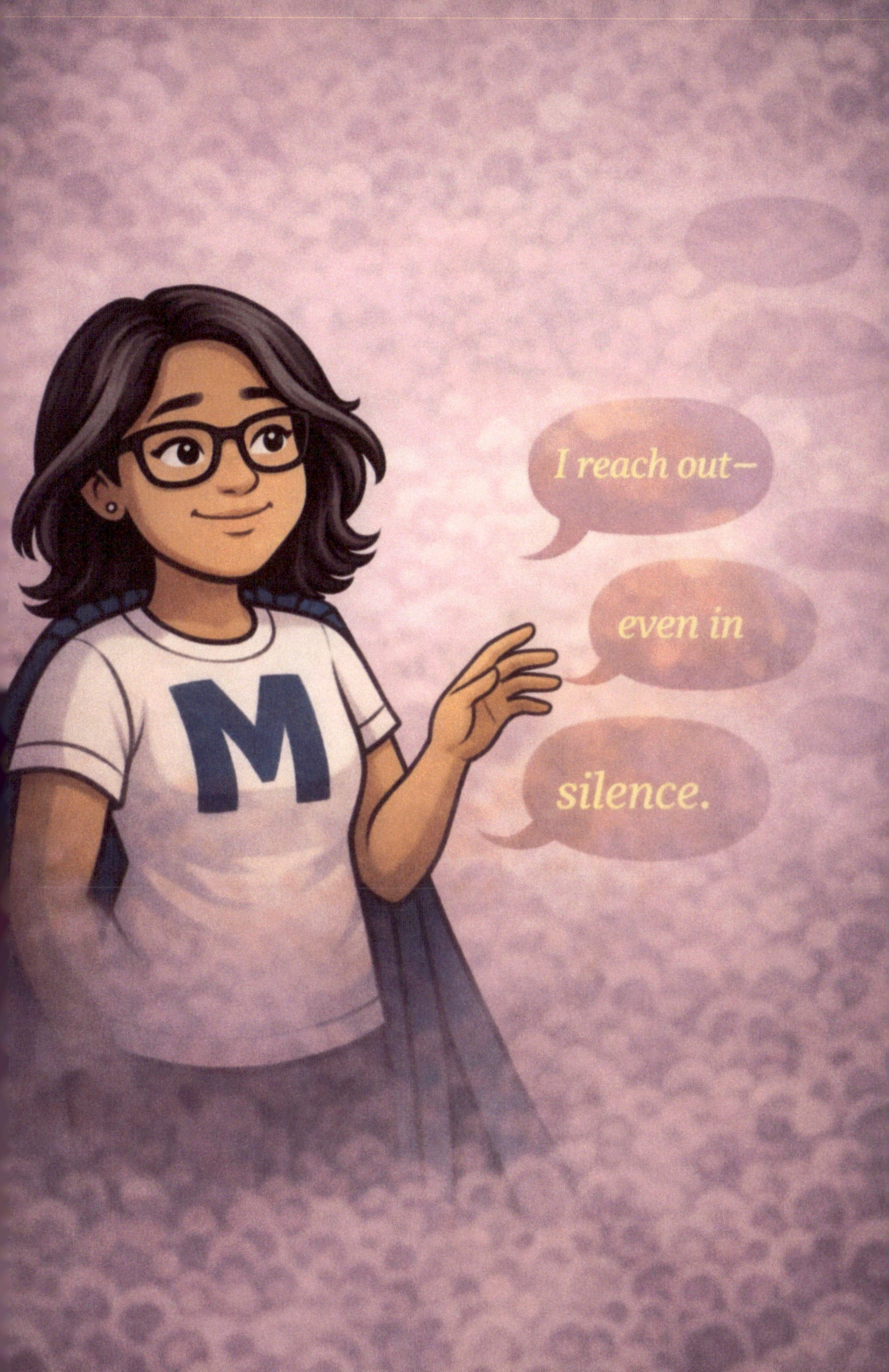
I reach out–
even in
silence.

You hold space for everyone else's feelings.

But when yours show up—
you tuck them away.

There's no room left.

But your feelings deserve space too.

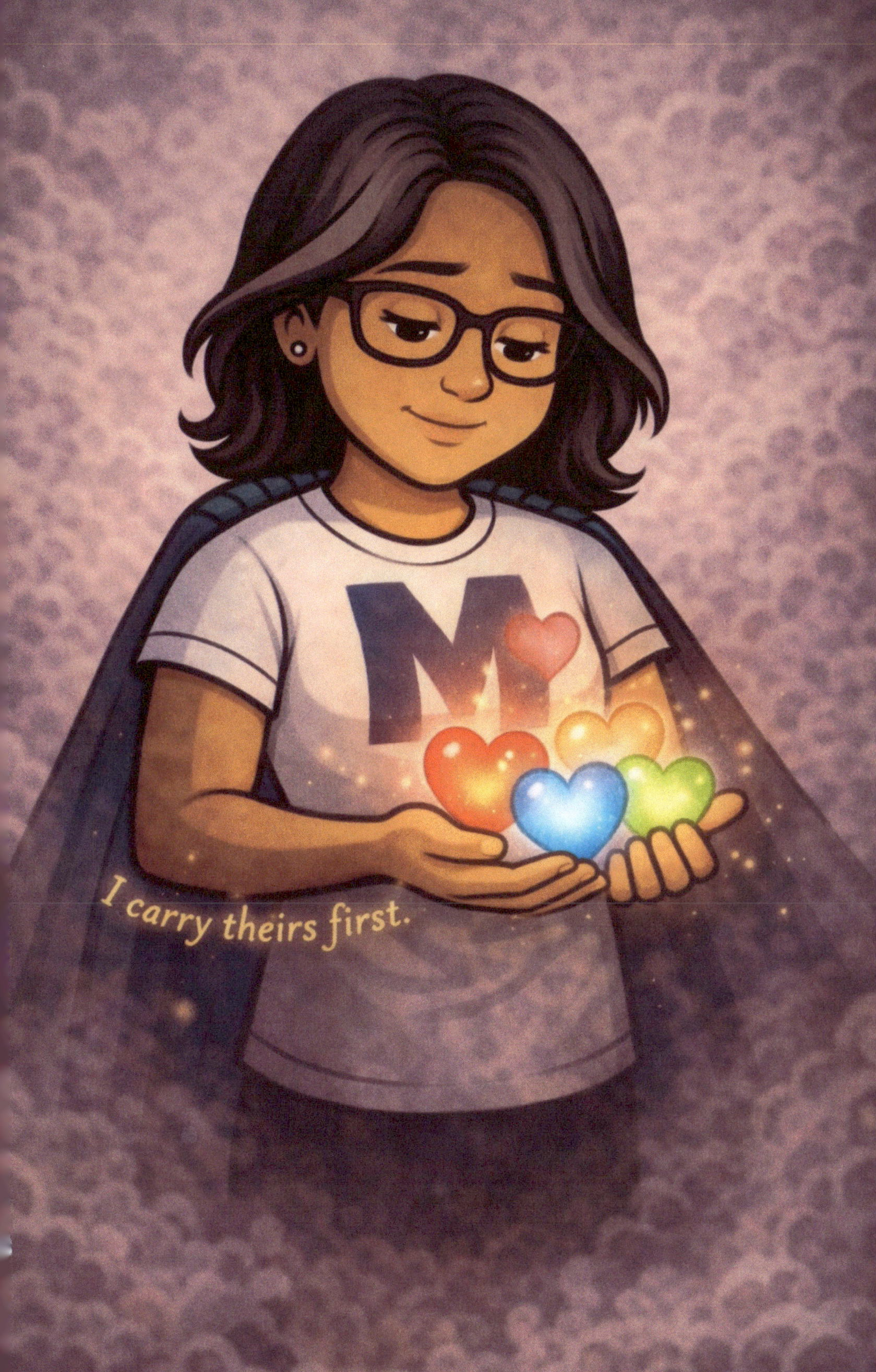
I carry theirs first.

You make things easier for others
without them ever realizing it was hard.

Because you plan, prepare, and carry
more than they see.

And that effort… it counts.

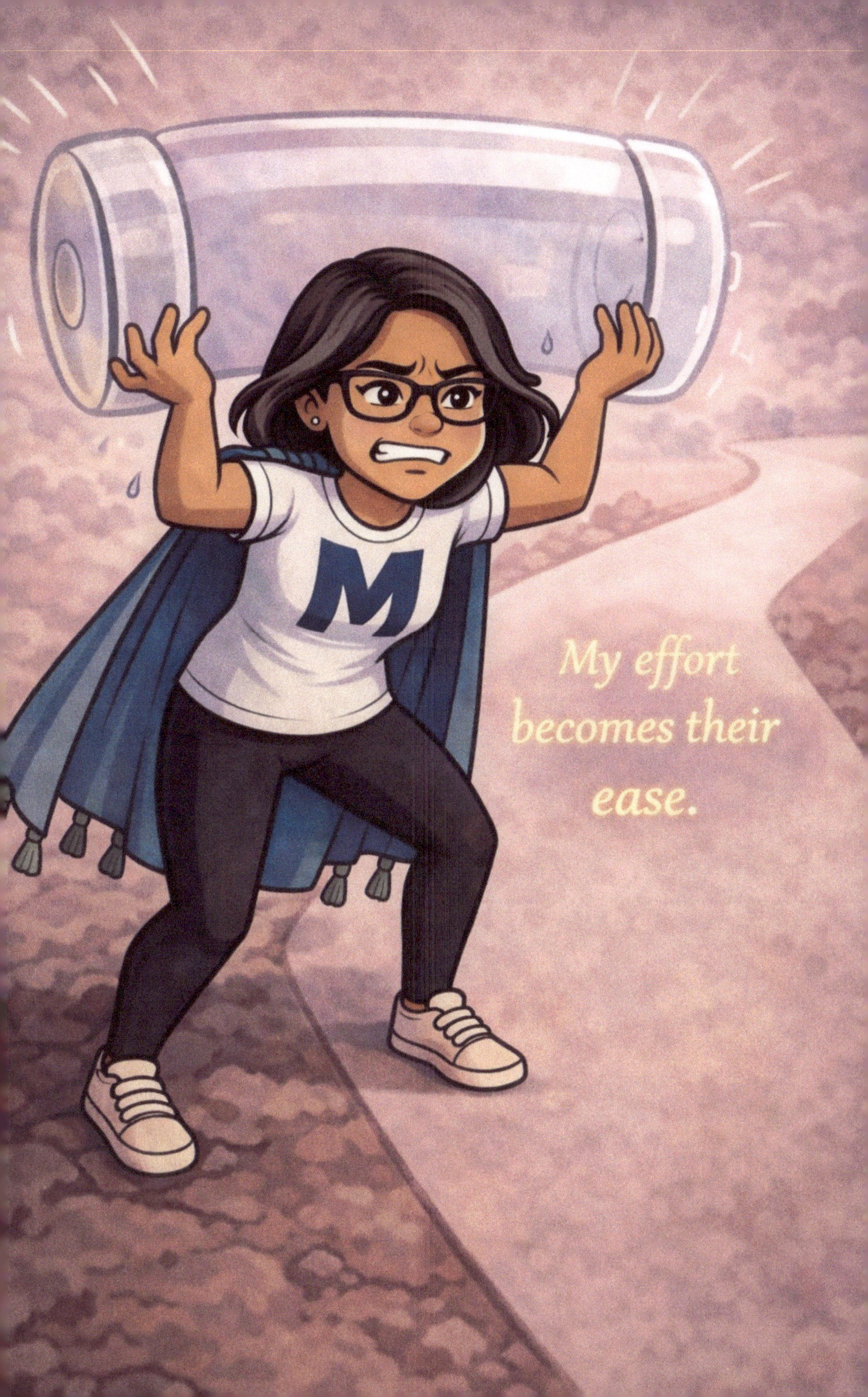
M
My effort
becomes their
ease.

You don't just do the work—
you think about the work.

Before it begins.
While it's happening.
Long after it's done.

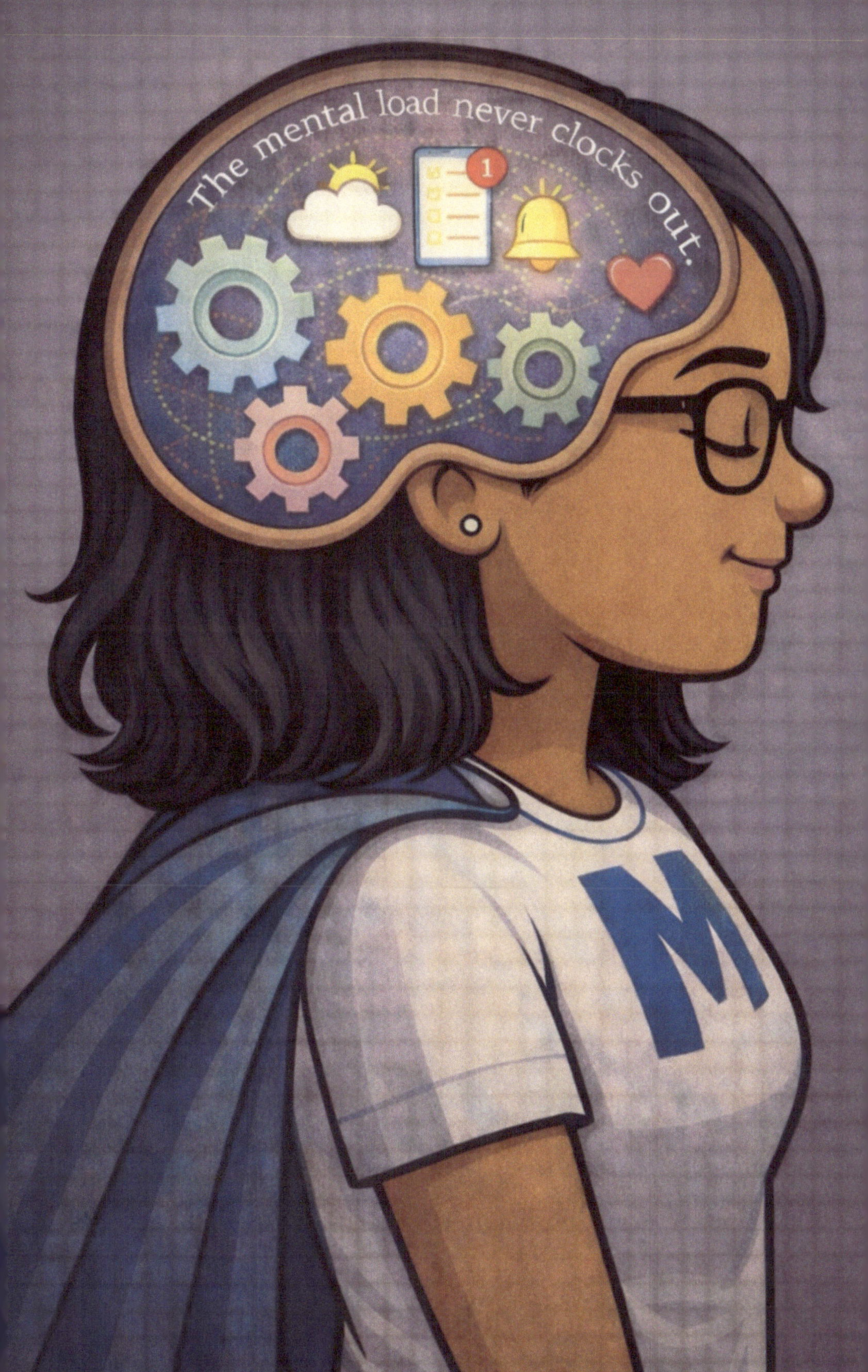
The mental load never clocks out.
M

You carry responsibility

no one ever clearly gave you.

It just... became yours.

Quietly. Gradually.

Until it was simply expected.

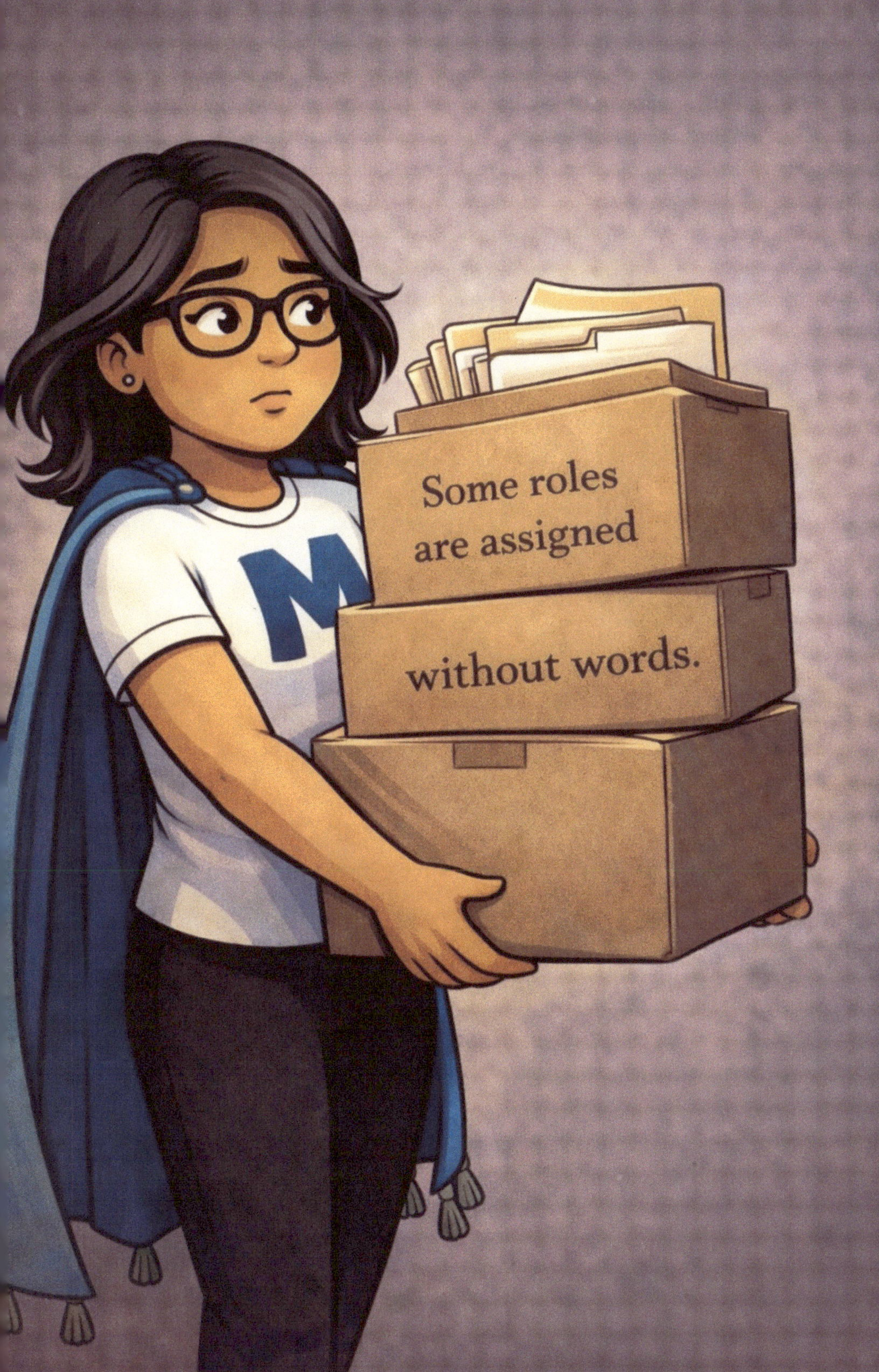
Some roles
are assigned
without words.

You keep things running so smoothly
that no one notices the effort.

No interruptions.
No gaps.

Because you’ve already filled them.

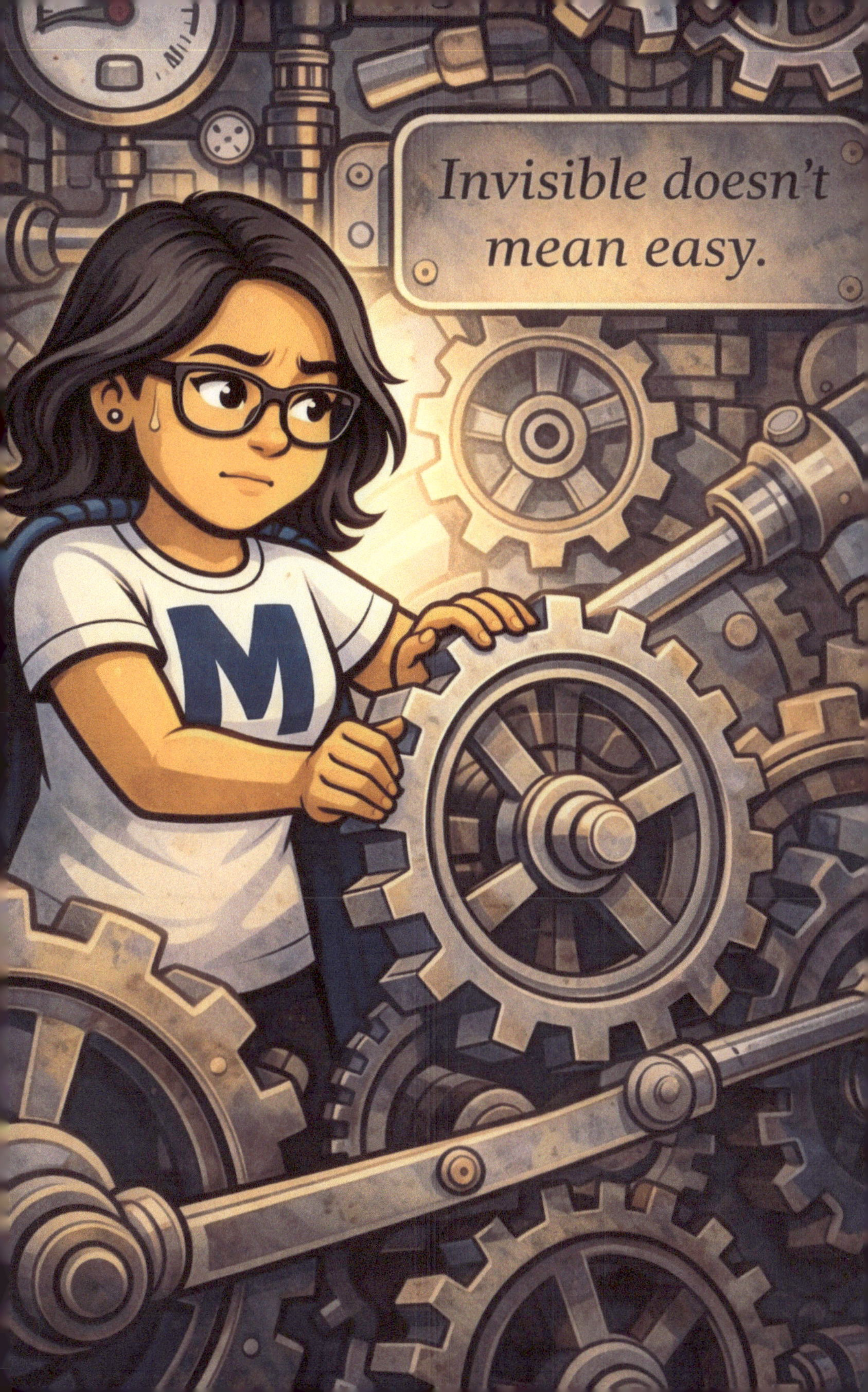
Invisible doesn't mean easy.

You feel guilty when you stop.

Even for a moment.

But resting isn't failing.
It's something you deserve too.

Rest feels unfamiliar.

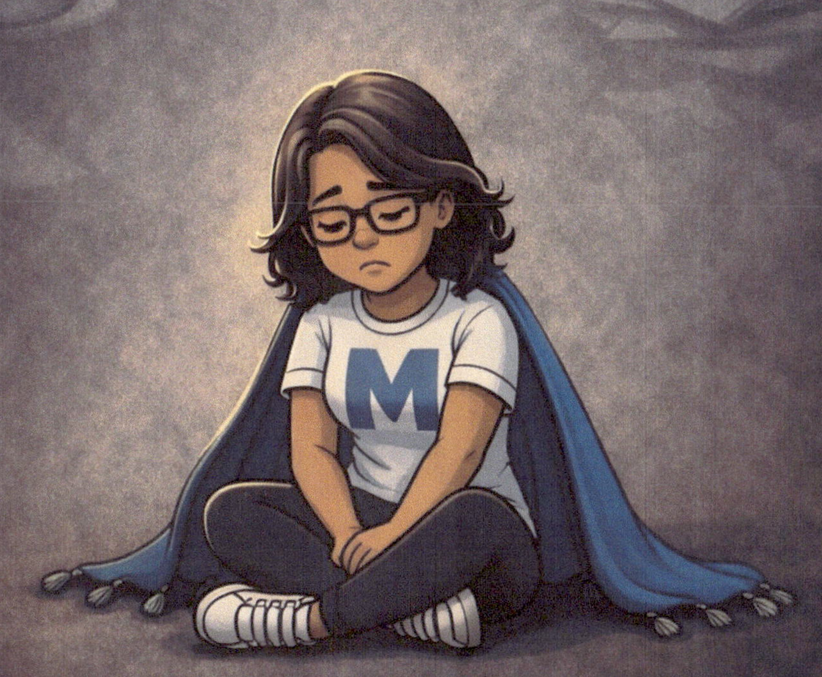

You’ve learned to hold it all together.

But no one asked
if you were okay doing that.

You just… did it.
Because someone had to.

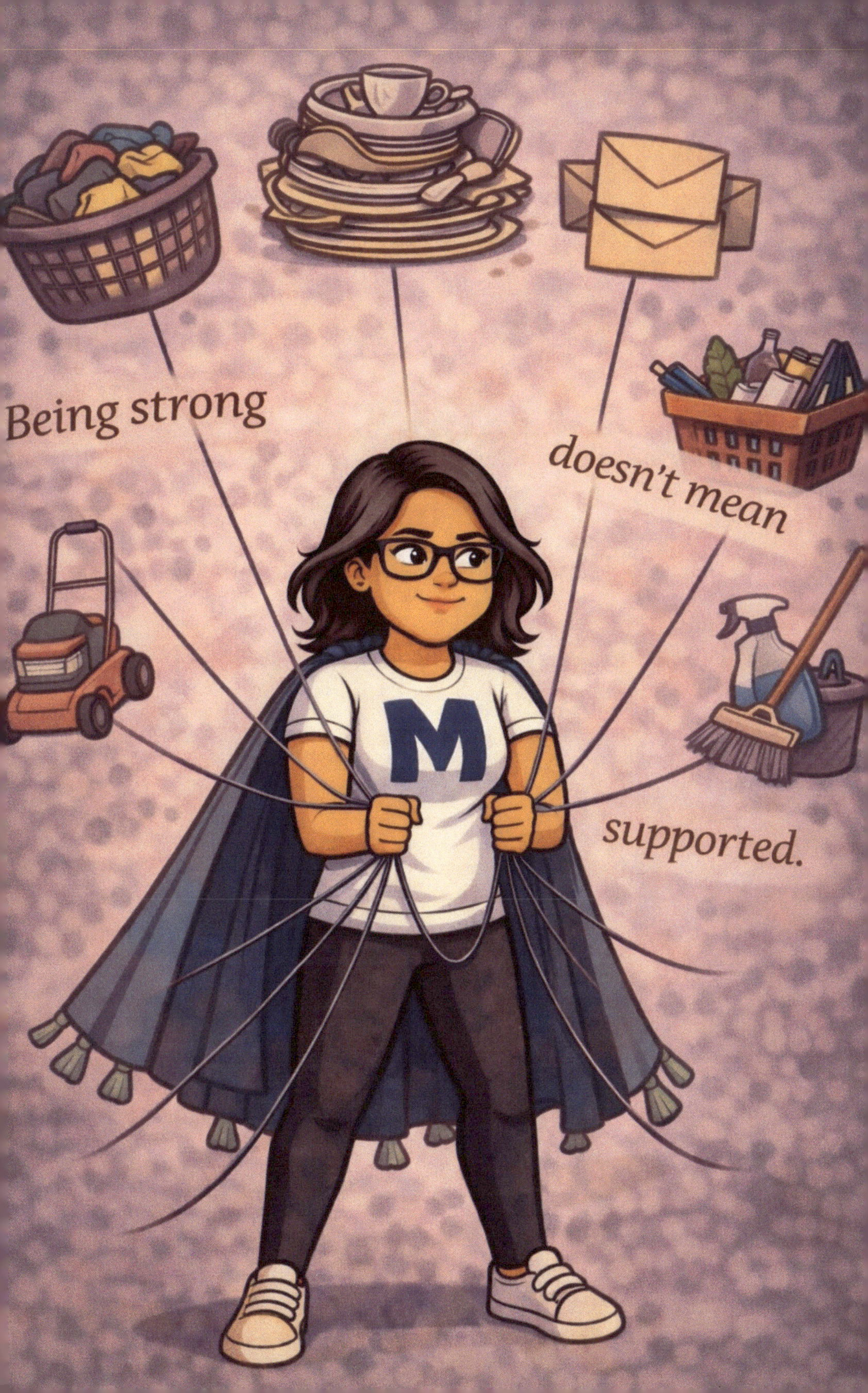
Being strong
doesn't mean
supported.

You became reliable.

Dependable.

The one who "just handles it."

And you've carried that role—

quietly, consistently, every day.

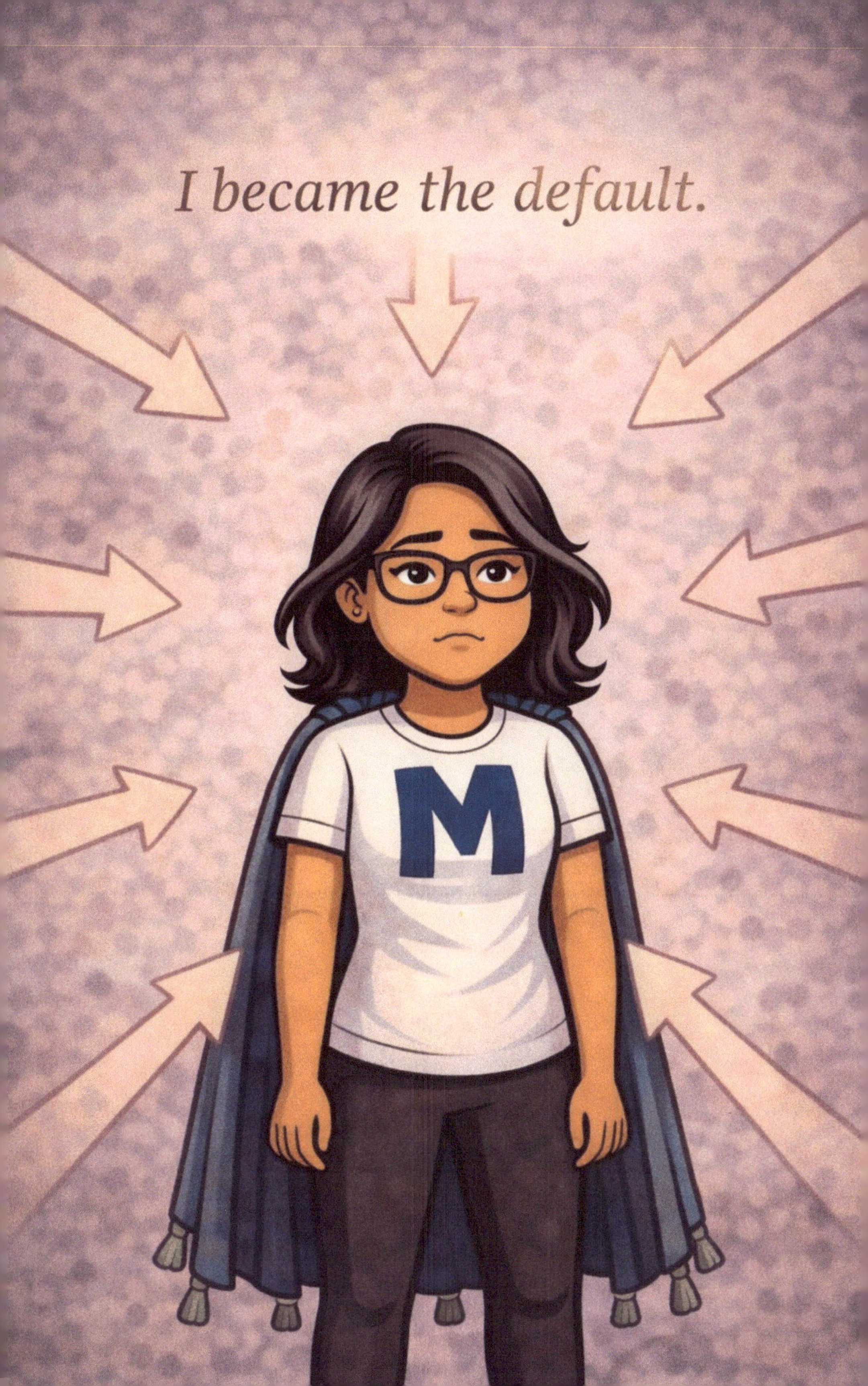
I became the default.
M

But being everything for everyone
was never meant to be your job alone.

It was never supposed to rest
entirely on you.

Somewhere along the way,
it just... did.

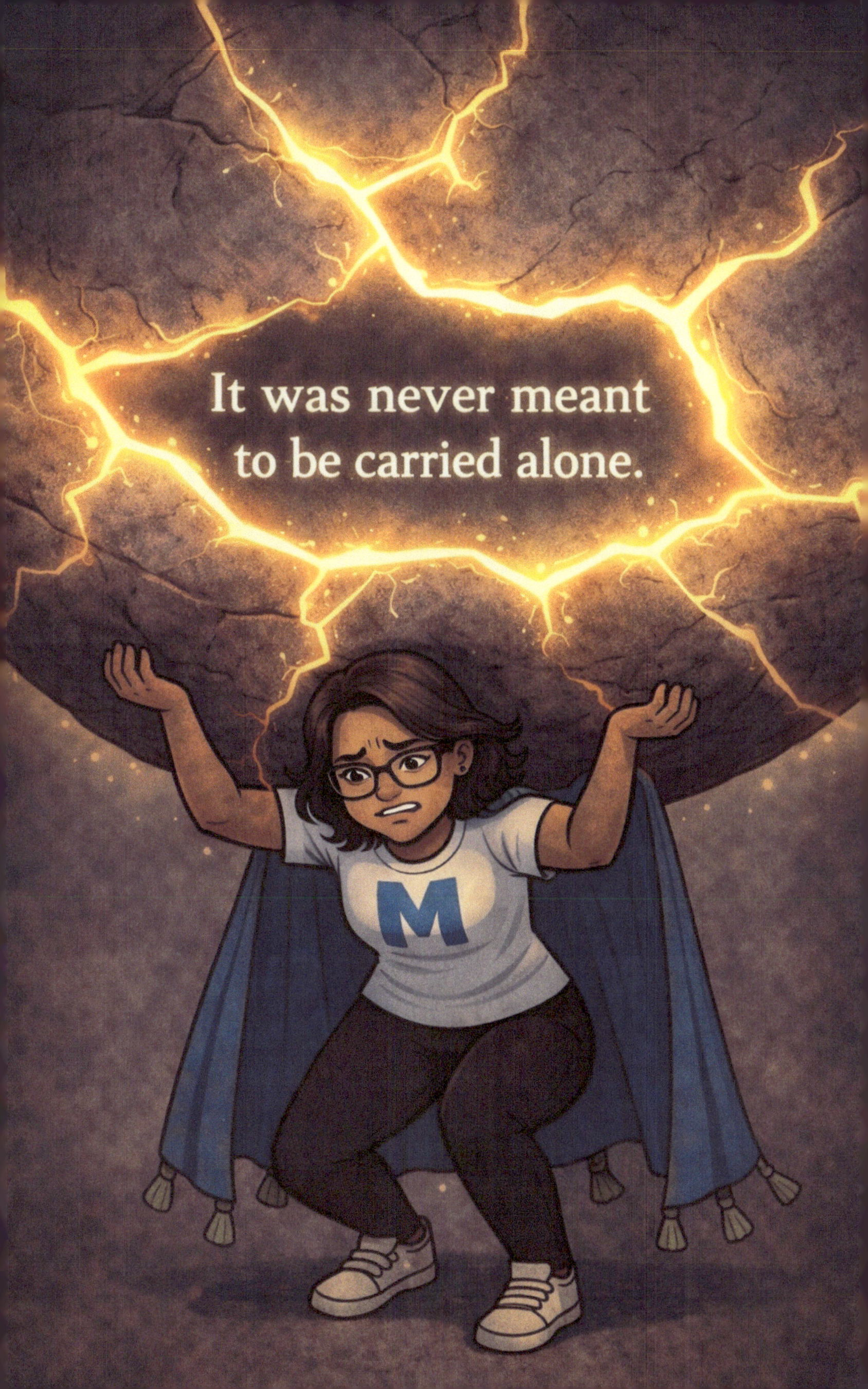
It was never meant
to be carried alone.
M

You are allowed to pause.

To not anticipate.

To not fix.

To not hold everything together.

You are allowed to rest your mind,

not just your body.

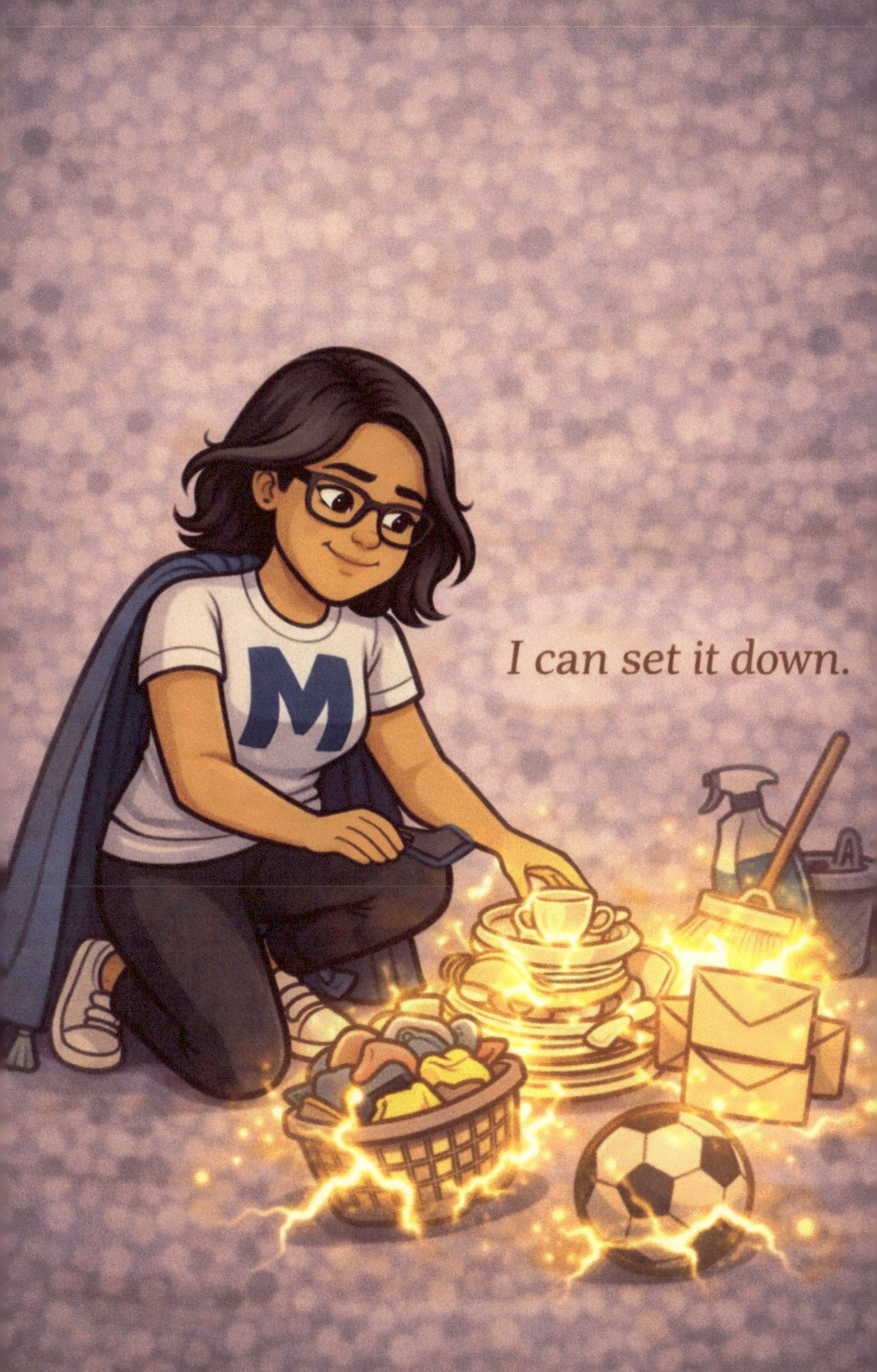
I can set it down.

You are allowed to be cared for
without earning it first.

Not after everything is done.
Not after you've given more.

Now. As you are.

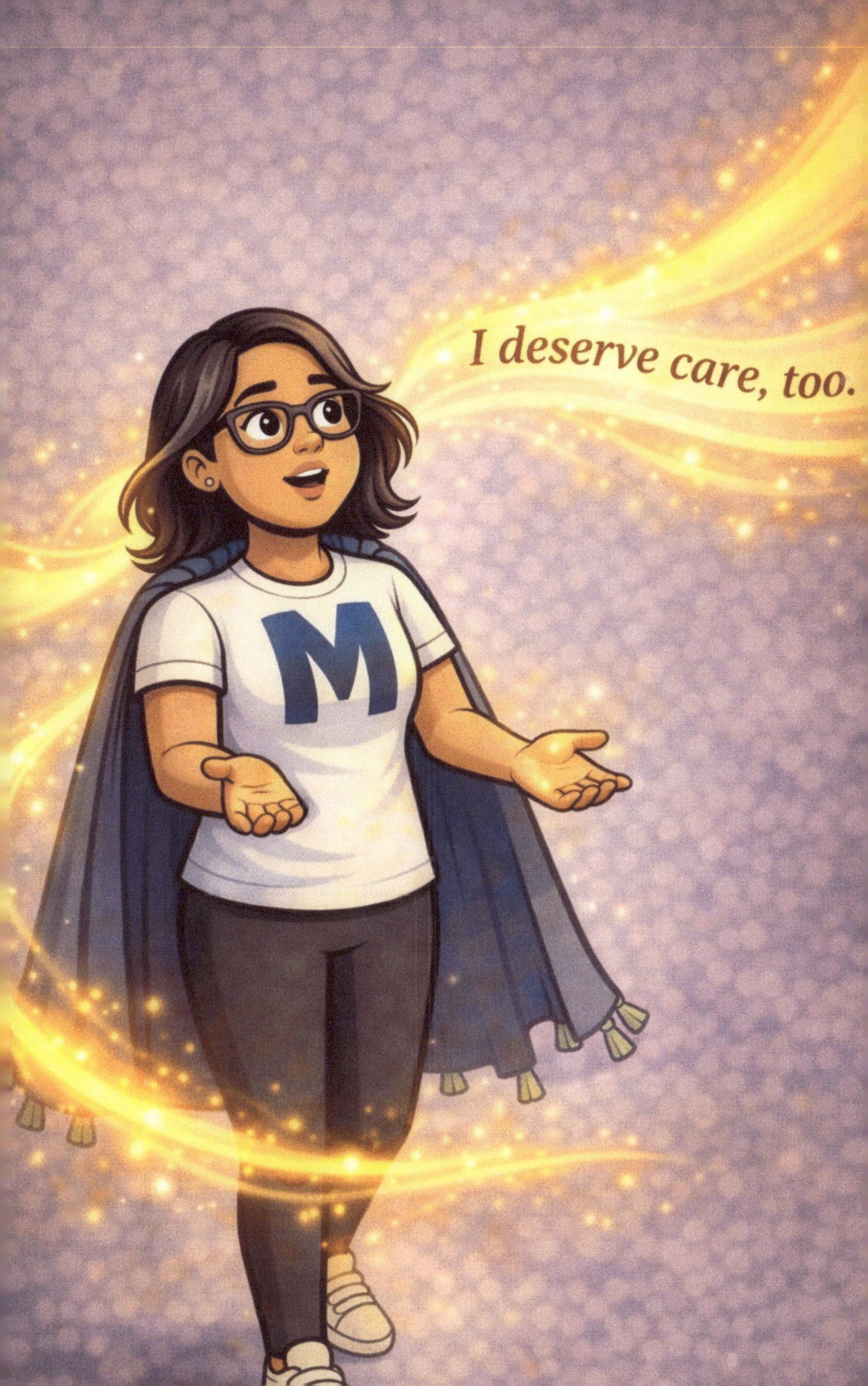
I deserve care, too.

You are not just what you manage.
You are not just what you hold.

You are a person
outside of what you carry.

I am more than the load.

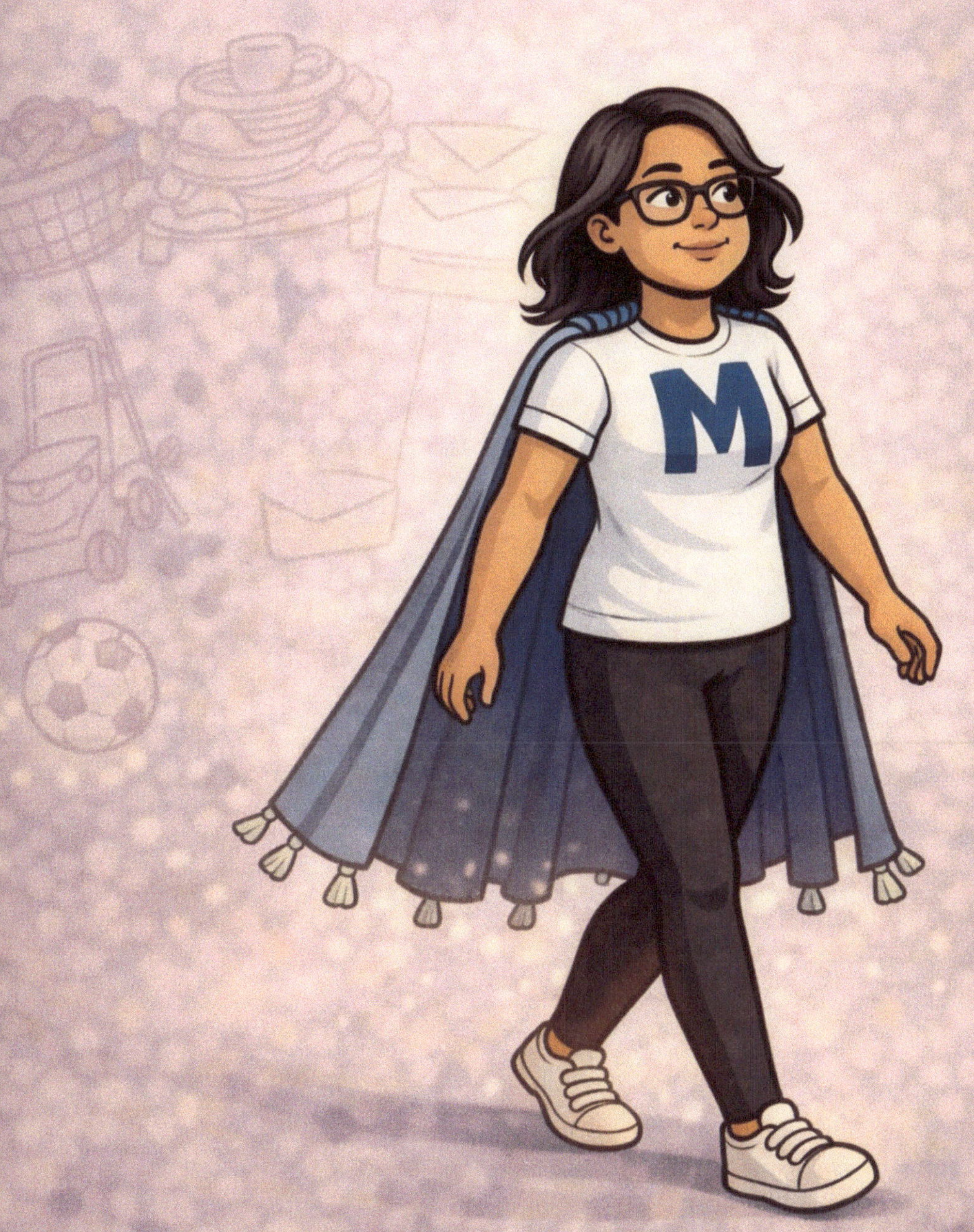

If no one has said it—
this work you've been doing,
this constant noticing, holding, remembering...

It matters.
But so do you.
You are allowed to take up space
without holding everything together.

You are allowed to rest
without everything falling apart.

And you are allowed
to be supported
in ways you've quietly given to others. ♡

I don't have to carry it all

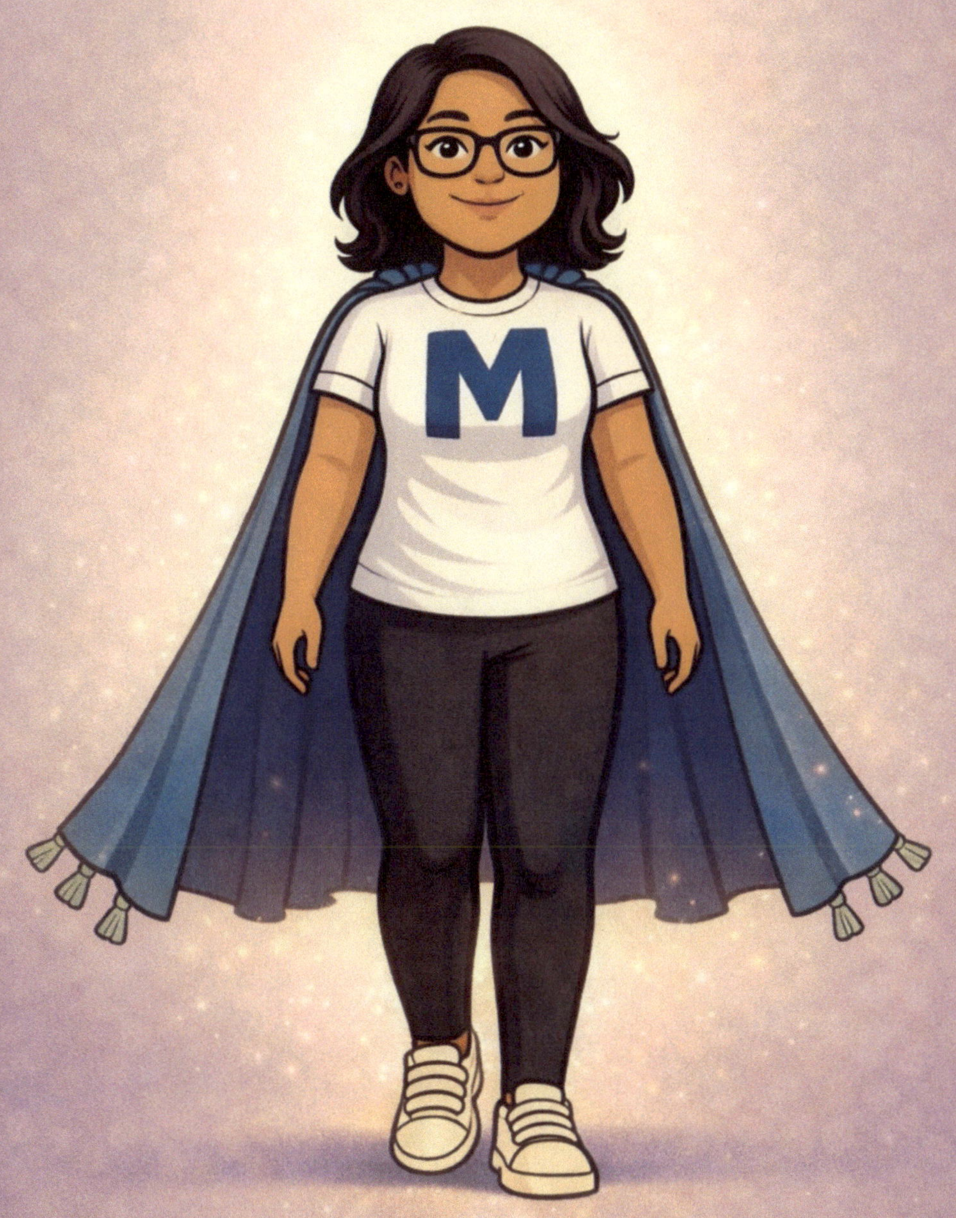

to be enough.

Also by MommyHooray

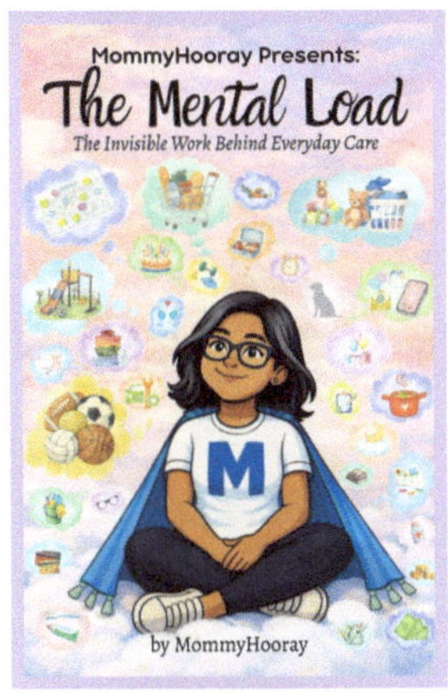

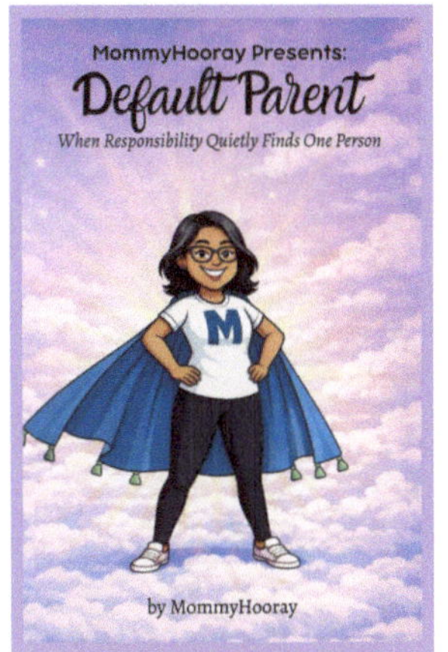

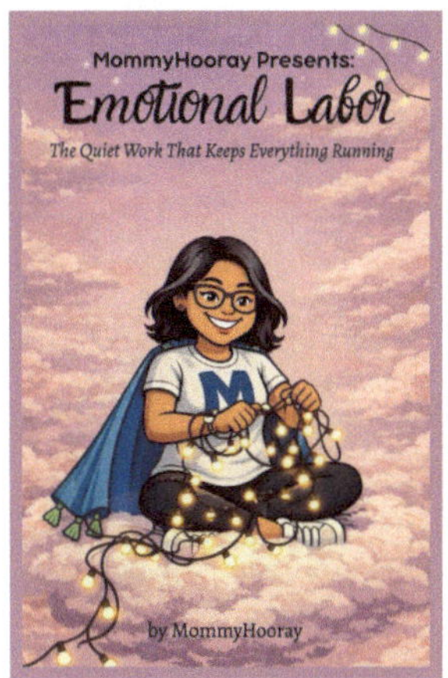

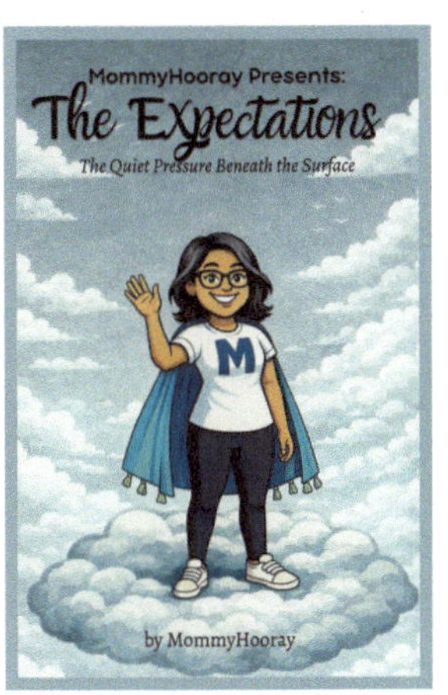

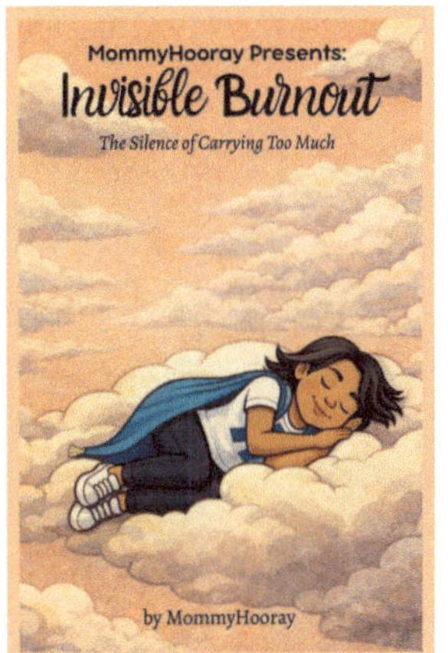

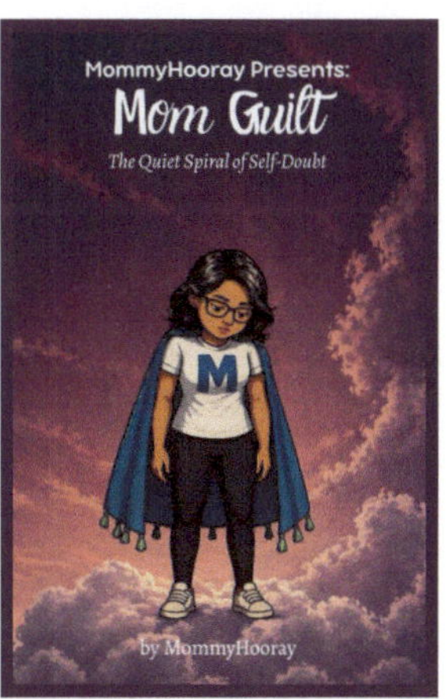

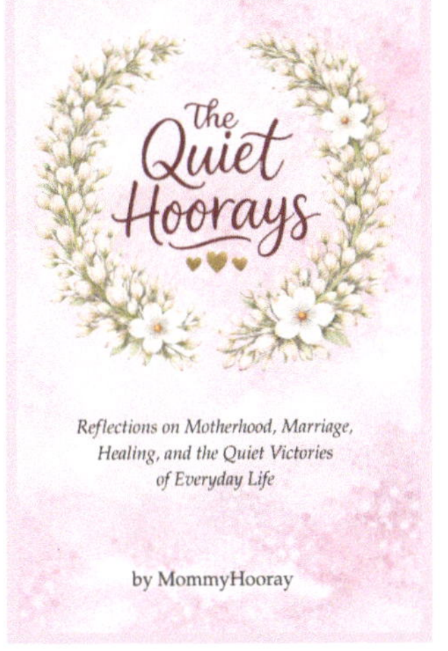

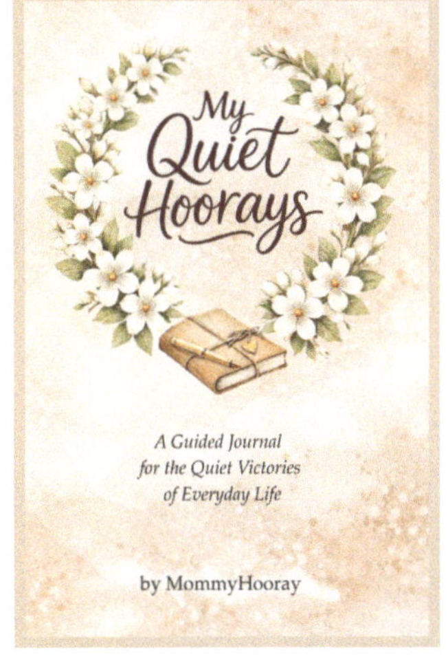

... and more!

From My Heart to Yours

Write something meaningful
for the person who will cherish this book, or for yourself.

Today's Date: ________________

May this page find you again, years from now.

www.ingramcontent.com/pod-product-compliance
Lightning Source LLC
LaVergne TN
LVHW052259100826
845147LV00001B/91

* 9 7 8 1 9 7 2 0 7 1 4 2 7 *